Infectious Diseases

Pocket Picture Guides
for Nurses

Infectious Diseases

W. Edmund Farrar
MD, FACP

Professor of Medicine and Microbiology,
Director, Infectious Diseases
and Immunology Division,
Medical University of South Carolina,
Charleston, South Carolina, USA

Harold P. Lambert
MD, FRCP

Professor of Microbial Diseases,
University of London,
Consultant Physician,
St. George's Hospital,
London, UK

Williams & Wilkins Baltimore London

Western Hemisphere distribution rights held by
Williams and Wilkins
428 East Preston Street
Baltimore, MD 21202, USA

ISBN 0-683-03042-6

Library of Congress Cataloging in Publication Data
Farrar, W. Edmund.
        Infectious diseases.
        (Pocket picture guides for nurses)
        1. Communicable diseases-Diagnosis-Atlases.
I. Lambert, Harold P. II. Title. III. Series.
[DNLM: 1. Communicable diseases-Diagnosis-Atlases
2. Communicable diseases-Diagnosis-Nursing texts.
WY17 F244i]
RC112.F37 1984   616.9′0475   83-5889

Project Editor: Fiona Carr
    Designer: Teresa Foster

Originated in Hong Kong by Imago Publishing Ltd.
Printed in Great Britain by W. S. Cowell Ltd.

Pocket Picture Guides
for Nurses

The purpose of this series is to provide essential visual
information about commonly encountered diseases in a
convenient practical and economic format. Each Pocket
Picture Guide covers an important area of day-to-day
clinical medicine. The main feature of these books is the
superbly photographed colour reproductions of typical
clinical appearances. Other visual diagnostic
information, such as X-rays, is included where
appropriate. Each illustration is fully explained by a
clearly written descriptive caption highlighting important
diagnostic features. Tables presenting other diagnostic
and differential diagnostic information are included
where appropriate. A comprehensive and carefully
compiled index makes each Pocket Picture Guide an easy
to use source of visual reference.

An extensive series is planned and other titles in the
initial group of Pocket Picture Guides are:

Rheumatic Diseases
Sexually Transmitted Diseases
Skin Diseases
Paediatrics

Contents

Introduction

In this book we have collected 164 figures to illustrate a wide variety of infectious diseases. Although most of these conditions are common in one or other parts of the world, we have also included a number of less familiar diseases which present characteristic appearances and have important therapeutic implications.

In addition to clinical photographs and radiographs, we have also included a number of pictures illustrating the results of easily available laboratory investigations. We hope that this collection will provide a valuable and easily used guide for both clinicians and laboratory workers.

A more extensive pictorial account of infectious diseases, including more than 700 photographs and line drawings with an integrated text, is available in "Infectious Diseases Illustrated" also by H. P. Lambert and W. E. Farrar.

Infections of the Upper Respiratory Tract

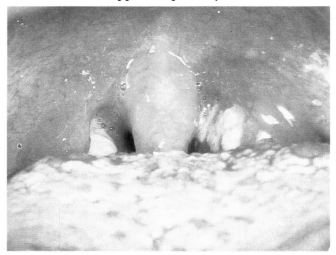

Fig. 1. Infectious mononucleosis. The tonsils are swollen and covered with uniform white exudate. The uvula looks swollen and the patient's speech is nasal.

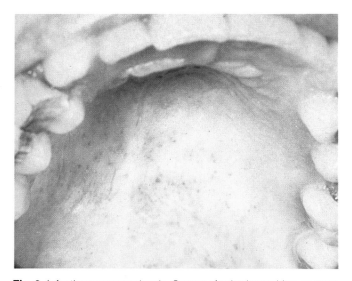

Fig. 2 Infectious mononucleosis. Groups of palatal petechiae, as seen in this picture, are common in infectious mononucleosis, but are not specific for this diagnosis, nor are they always seen even in severe forms of this illness.

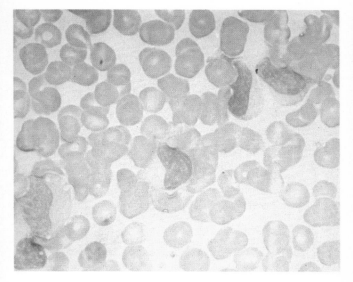

Fig. 3 Infectious mononucleosis. Blood film showing atypical lymphocytes. These are larger than normal lymphocytes with a higher ratio of cytoplasm to nucleus. The cytoplasm is basophilic and the nucleus indented or lobulated.

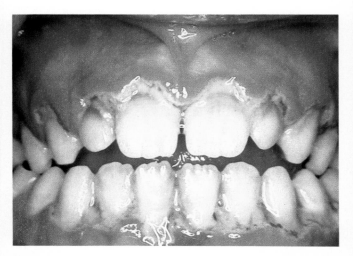

Fig. 4 Acute ulcerative gingivitis (Vincent's infection). Ulceration of the gingival margin is associated with accumulation of bacterial plaque. The gums are swollen with areas of necrosis and the breath fetid. *Borrelia vincentii* (a spirillary organism) and fusiform anaerobic bacteria are found in the plaque.

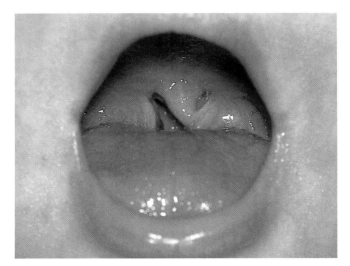

Fig. 5 Scarlet fever. The throat is generally red and the tonsils swollen and dark red with spots of exudate. If the organism is a producer of the erythrogenic toxin, the local signs are accompanied by the punctate erythematous rash of scarlet fever (see Fig. 64).

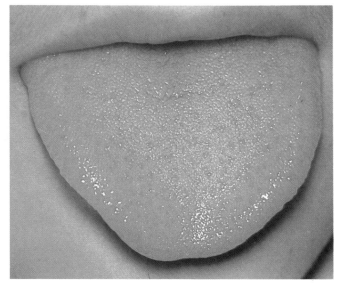

Fig. 6 Scarlet fever. In the early stages there is a dense white coating. Later this peels off leaving a raw red surface, with prominent follicles, the 'strawberry tongue'.

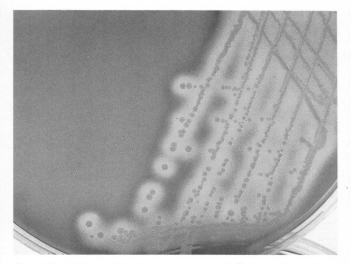

Fig. 7 Scarlet fever (*Streptococcus pyogenes*). The causal organism grows on blood agar giving small colonies surrounded by a clear zone in which the blood has been completely lysed (β haemolysis).

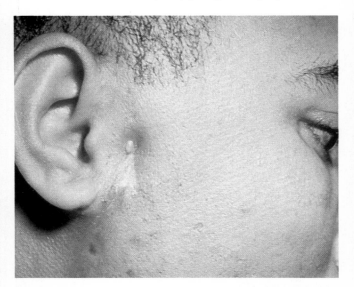

Fig. 8 Actinomycosis. A common site is the cervicofacial region, arising from a dental source. The initial swelling is followed by a chronic discharging sinus, as seen in this picture. Other sites of actinomycosis are the lungs and thoracic wall, and the ileocaecal region. By courtesy of Dr. T. F. Sellers, Jr.

4

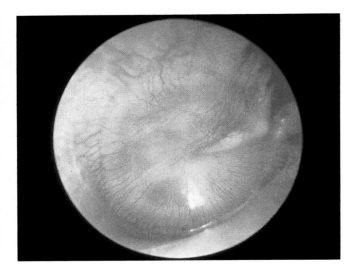

Fig. 9 Otitis media. In the early stages the redness is most prominent in the region of the malleus. The most common bacterial causes are *Streptococcus pneumoniae* and *Haemophilus influenzae,* with *Streptococcus pyogenes* less commonly found. A small proportion of cases are caused by *Neisseria catarrhalis*. By courtesy of Dr. M. Chaput de Saintonge.

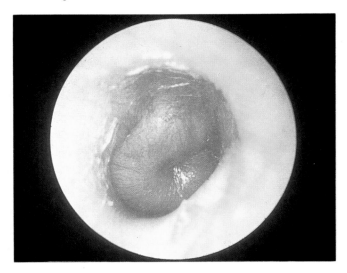

Fig. 10 Acute otitis media. Advanced stage with bulging drum. These appearances are seen just before the drum perforates. By courtesy of Dr. M. Chaput de Saintonge.

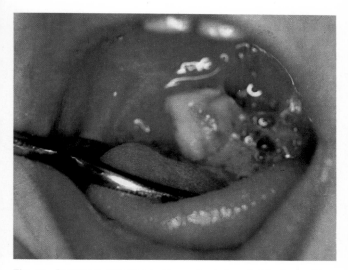

Fig. 11 Diphtheria. Infection by *Corynebacterium diphtheriae* is still common in some developing countries. Clinical manifestations vary between carrier state and life-threatening illness. This photograph shows severe diphtheria with gross swelling and congestion of the whole pharynx and tonsillar area. Dirty white exudate covers both tonsils and is spreading to the posterior pharyngeal wall. By courtesy of Dr. I. Zamiri.

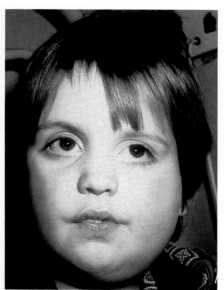

Fig 12 Mumps. Bilateral non-suppurative parotitis is the characteristic syndrome. Submandibular gland enlargement often follows that of the parotids. The common complications of mumps are meningoencephalitis, pancreatitis and, in the post-pubertal male, orchitis. By courtesy of Dr. G. D. W. McKendrick.

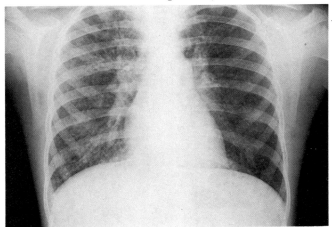

Fig. 13 Viral pneumonia. Some viruses, such as influenza, can cause pneumonia in the normal host while others, such as cytomegalovirus cause lung disease mainly in the immunosuppressed. The radiograph, as here, usually shows diffuse bilateral abnormalities and this appearance could be caused by a number of different viral and other pathogens.

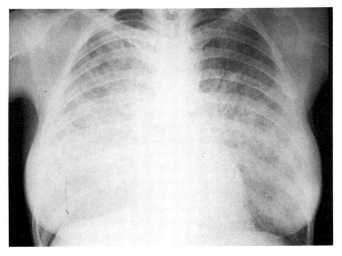

Fig. 14 Viral pneumonia – varicella. This may occur in previously healthy patients or in the immunosuppressed. The patient may be very ill with severe hypoxia. The individual nodular shadows are sometimes larger than in this example, and recovery is sometimes followed by calcification in the residual nodules.

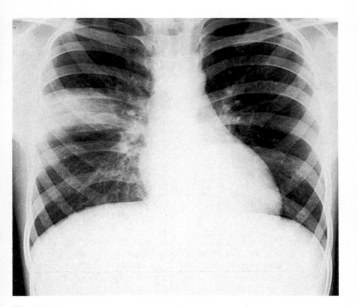

Fig. 15 Pneumococcal pneumonia is characterized by its sudden onset accompanied by rigors, high fever, pleural pain, rusty sputum and neutrophilia. This 'classical' form is now uncommon in wealthier countries. Nevertheless, *Streptococcus pneumoniae* remains the dominant cause of community-acquired pneumonia and is common also in nosocomial pneumonia. Consolidation may involve a complete lobe or, as in this radiograph, a segment.

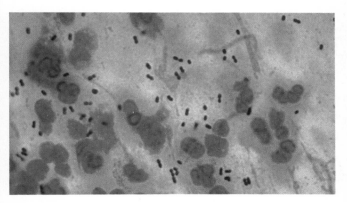

Fig. 16 Pneumococcal pneumonia. A Gram stain film of the sputum shows pneumococci seen mostly as lanceolate diplococci. Other organisms are seen among the leucocytes but pneumococci predominate and are likely to represent the significant pathogen. By courtesy of Dr. J. R. Cantey.

8

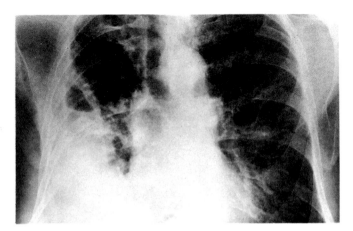

Fig. 17 Empyema. Transient pleural effusion is common in pneumonia and sometimes the effusion becomes purulent. This radiograph shows a large right pleural effusion with an air-fluid level. This pyopneumothorax or hydropneumothorax could result from insertion of air during aspiration or from the formation of a bronchopleural fistula.

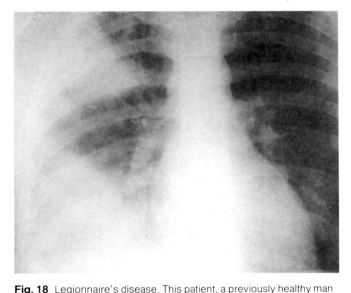

Fig. 18 Legionnaire's disease. This patient, a previously healthy man aged 43 years, became infected in Spain. He had a stormy course with prolonged high fever, severe pneumonia and, in the early stages, diarrhoea and a toxic confusional state. This chest radiograph shows his predominantly right lower and right upper lobe pneumonia. *Legionella pneumonophila* infection was proved serologically.

9

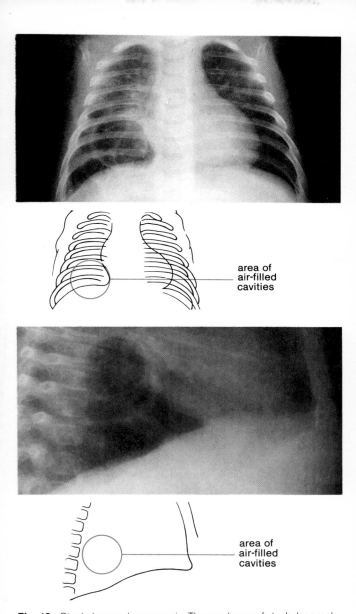

area of
air-filled
cavities

area of
air-filled
cavities

Fig. 19 Staphylococcal pneumonia. The syndrome of staphylococcal pneumonia in childhood is characterized by the formation of pneumatocoeles as seen in these radiographs, which may form abscesses and have a tendency to rupture to give a staphylococcal pyopneumothorax.

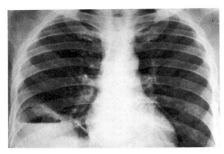

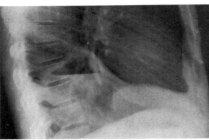

Fig. 20 Lung abscess. Pulmonary suppuration occurs usually following aspiration or in association with bronchial obstruction. Abscesses can develop as a complication of pneumonia, for example, in that caused by *Klebsiella pneumoniae,* and multiple abscesses of blood-borne origin occur in some forms of septicaemia, for example, in staphylococcal septicaemia in drug addicts. These radiographs show a single large abscess in the right lower lobe.

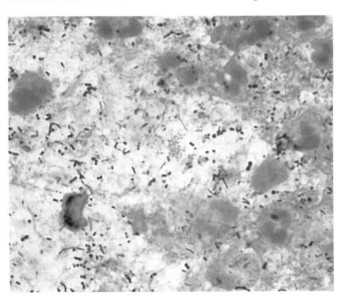

Fig. 21 Lung abscess. The flora in lung abscesses is polymicrobial, often with a mixture of aerobes and anaerobes. This Gram stain film of pus from a lung abscess shows Gram-positive cocci and variable Gram-positive and Gram-negative rods. By courtesy of Dr. J. R. Cantey.

11

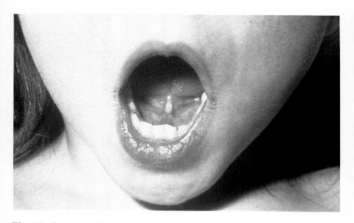

Fig. 22 Pertussis. The main features of this infection are paroxysmal cough often accompanied by vomiting and whooping. Infants often have apnoeic attacks, and are also more liable to develop pneumonia than are older children. Sometimes the severe prolonged cough gives rise to complications such as conjunctival haemorrhages (see Fig. 118) or, as in this patient, a frenal ulcer caused by the frequent gagging and vomiting. By courtesy of Dr. G. D. W. McKendrick.

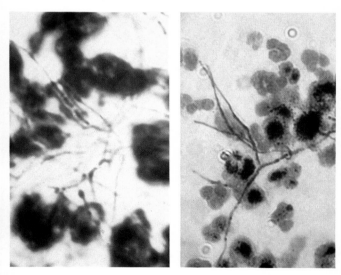

Fig. 23 Pulmonary nocardiosis. *Nocardia asteroides* is the usual species found in man, causing pulmonary consolidation, abscess, and empyema especially in immunocompromised patients. The organisms can be seen by Ziehl-Neelsen or Gram staining as irregular or beaded narrow branching filaments. By courtesy of Dr. T. F. Sellers, Jr. (left) and Dr. H. P. Holley, Jr. (right).

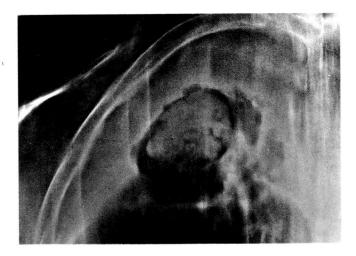

Fig. 24 Aspergillosis. This fungus may cause transient pulmonary infiltrates with eosinophilia in allergic subjects, or life-threatening pneumonia in the immunosuppressed. The fungus may also grow locally in areas of lung affected by chronic diseases such as tuberculosis, bronchiectasis or sarcoidosis. In this tomogram the aspergilloma (fungus ball) is outlined by air shadow in an old tuberculous cavity.

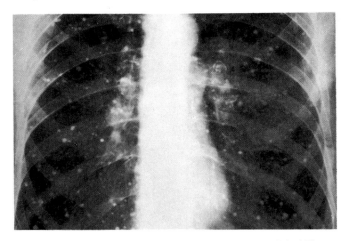

Fig. 25 Histoplasmosis. Primary infection is usually subclinical. The acute forms include multifocal lung shadows with enlarged hilar nodes; some patients develop erythema nodosum or erythema multiforme. Another acute variety presents as diffuse miliary shadowing and, when this heals, the radiograph shows multiple small areas of calcification. By courtesy of Dr. M. Pearson.

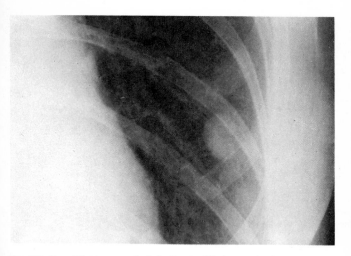

Fig. 26 Coccidioidomycosis. Infection by this fungus is also usually subclinical, although some patients have respiratory symptoms and even pneumonia. Again, erythema nodosum or erythema multiforme may accompany primary infection. Chronic cavitating pulmonary disease may follow, but a solitary lung nodule or 'coin' lesion is a more common sequel. This may calcify in the course of time.

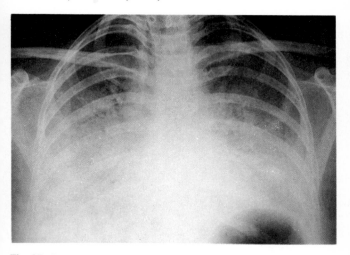

Fig. 27 *Pneumocystis carinii.* This is probably a common protozoal infection of man. It causes pneumonia in children suffering from severe malnutrition and in patients with severe immunosuppression, especially those receiving steroids or other immunosuppressive drugs. This radiograph shows the more common appearance of extensive 'ground-glass' opacities in both lower zones.

Infections of the Central Nervous System

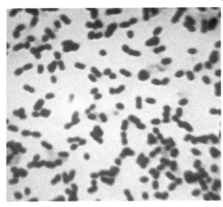

Fig. 28
Pneumococcal meningitis. In this Gram stain of cerebrospinal fluid, large numbers of Gram-positive diplococci are seen, with only a few fragments of degenerating polymorphonuclear leucocytes. By courtesy of Dr. T. F. Sellers, Jr.

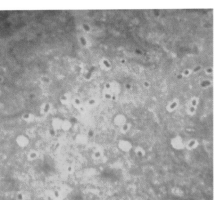

Fig. 29 *Klebsiella pneumoniae* meningitis. This Gram stain of cerebrospinal fluid shows many heavily encapsulated Gram-negative bacilli and much proteinaceous material. By courtesy of Dr. V. E. Del Bene.

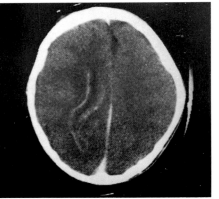

Fig. 30 Bacterial meningitis. This computerized tomographic (CT) scan shows enhancement of the ependyma of the right lateral ventricle, as seen in ventriculitis complicating bacterial meningitis. By courtesy of Dr. G. D. Hungerford.

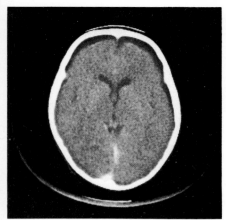

Fig. 31 Bacterial meningitis. Subdural effusion in the frontal region is seen in this CT scan from a patient with meningitis due to *Haemophilus influenzae*. By courtesy of Dr. G. D. Hungerford.

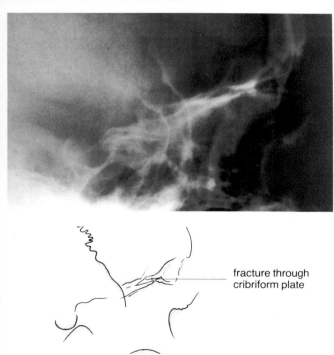

fracture through cribriform plate

Fig. 32 Recurrent bacterial meningitis. This lateral skull film shows a fracture through the cribriform plate. Most cases of recurrent bacterial meningitis are due to *Streptococcus pneumoniae,* but infections due to *Haemophilus influenzae* or *Neisseria meningitidis* are occasionally seen. By courtesy of Dr. G. D. Hungerford.

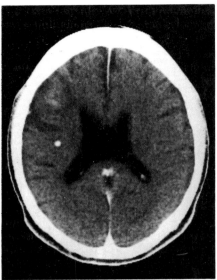

Fig. 33 Cryptococcal meningitis. Computerized tomography often reveals discrete, clinically silent lesions within the brain substance. This scan shows a calcified granuloma in the right parietal lobe. Normal vascular enhancement is seen. By courtesy of G. D. Hungerford.

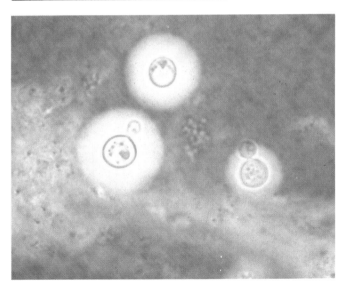

Fig. 34 Cryptococcal meningitis. The heavily encapsulated cells of *Cryptococcus neoformans* may often be identified in the centrifugal sediment of cerebrospinal fluid after a drop of India ink has been added. Note the highly refractile cell wall and internal structure, which distinguish these yeast cells from lymphocytes. By courtesy of A. E. Prevost.

17

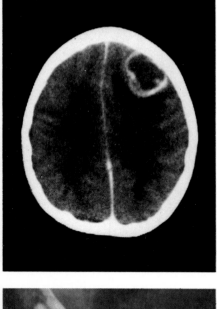

Fig. 35 Brain abscess. Infection is usually due to anaerobic bacteria, or a combination of anaerobic and aerobic bacteria, except when it occurs as a complication of bacterial endocarditis. This CT scan shows the typical appearance of a brain abscess in the left frontal lobe with enhancement of the capsule. The uniform thin wall is characteristic of abscess rather than tumour . By courtesy of Dr. G. D. Hungerford.

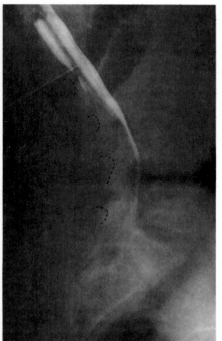

Fig. 36 Spinal epidural abscess. This lumbar myelogram shows anterior displacement of the column of contrast material by a posterior epidural abscess. By courtesy of Dr. G. D. Hungerford.

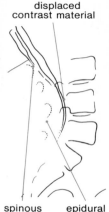

displaced
contrast material

spinous
process

epidural
abscess

18

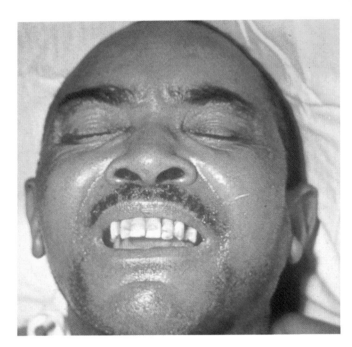

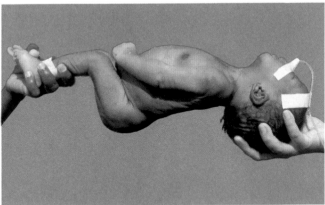

Fig. 37 Tetanus. The disease is due to the action of toxin (tetanospasmin) produced by *Clostridium tetani* on synapses within the central nervous system. The characteristic clinical manifestations are trismus ('lockjaw') and generalized muscle spasms. *Risus sardonicus,* the 'sardonic smile', is caused by spasm of the facial muscles and is a feature of tetanus in older children and adults. Opisthotonus, due to intense contraction of the paravertebral muscles, is seen most commonly in neonatal tetanus. By courtesy of Dr. T. F. Sellers, Jr.

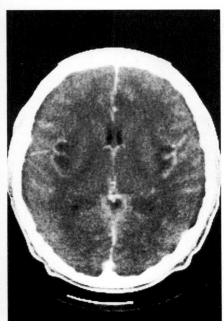

Fig. 38 *Herpes simplex* encephalitis. CT scanning almost always reveals focal abnormalities in patients with this infection. This scan shows the characteristic feature of low density lesions with associated gyral enhancement in the region of the Sylvian fissures. By courtesy of Dr. G. D. Hungerford.

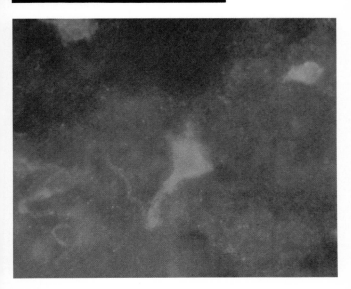

Fig. 39 *Herpes simplex* encephalitis. In this brain biopsy stained by immunofluorescence the neurons heavily infected with herpes simplex virus are stained a bright green. By courtesy of Dr. S. Fisher-Hoch.

Cutaneous Manifestations of Viral Infection

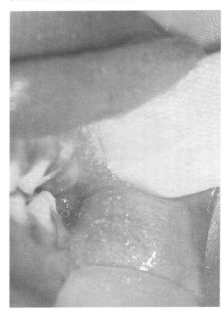

Fig. 40 Measles. Koplik's spots are seen on the buccal mucosa about a day before the rash appears and they remain for two or three days. They are minute white spots on an erythematous base, best seen in the lower buccal groove. They are also sometimes seen on the conjunctiva.

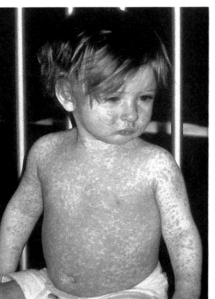

Fig. 41 Measles. This is a very characteristic picture. A miserable child, with a blotchy rash, runny nose and bleary eyes. The rash is denser on the face than on the trunk and has a purple tinge. In fair-skinned patients, after the severe illness has subsided, there is much 'staining' of the areas affected by the rash. This purpuric rash lasts a few more days but leaves no sequelae.

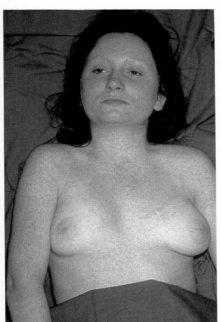

Fig. 42 Rubella. The rash of rubella consists of discrete pink macules, although the facial eruption is often confluent. The face and trunk are affected most on the first day and the rash then spreads downwards and peripherally. Generalized lymphadenopathy precedes and accompanies the rash. The features of rubella vary greatly and clinical diagnosis is unreliable.

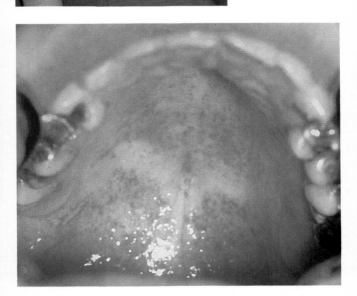

Fig. 43 Rubella. Red spots are often seen on the palate (Forchheimer spots); in this patient they were exceptionally profuse.

22

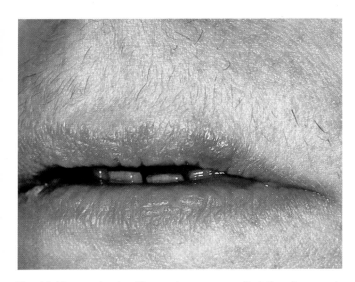

Fig. 44 Herpes simplex. The most common manifestation of recurrent infection is the cold sore, seen on the mucocutaneous margin. Sometimes recurrent herpes simplex is found at other sites. The early appearance, seen in this photograph, is of a localized swelling which soon reveals itself as a cluster of closely packed vesicles.

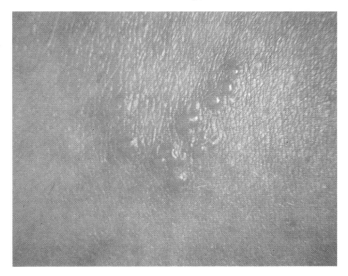

Fig. 45 Herpes simplex. Here, in more fully developed form than in the previous slide, is the characteristic irregularly grouped cluster of small vesicles. By courtesy of Dr. V. E. Del Bene.

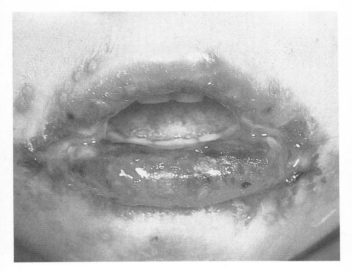

Fig. 46 Herpes simplex. Acute gingivostomatitis is a common consequence of primary infection in small children. The tongue, lips, and buccal mucosa are red with shallow ulcers filled with white exudate. The skin may be normal but in some children the vesicular lesions of herpes appear on the skin around the mouth.

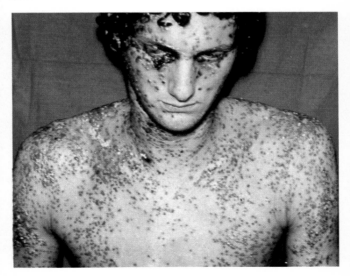

Fig. 47 Eczema herpeticum. Patients with eczema tend to develop widespread dissemination of herpetic skin lesions. The eruption is most dense in the eczematous areas but is not confined to them.

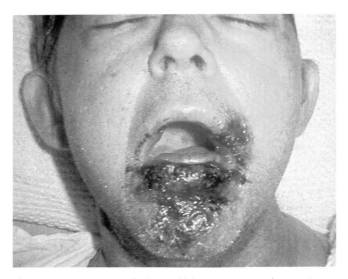

Fig. 48 Herpes simplex. Patients with immunosuppression are at special risk from this virus. This patient with leukaemia developed severe lesions with necrosis of the skin. By courtesy of Dr. V. E. Del Bene.

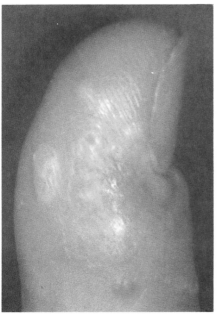

Fig. 49 Herpetic whitlow. This is seen after accidental inoculation with herpes simplex virus, and thumb-sucking children sometimes develop herpetic paronychia when they have oral herpes. The lesion may look just like a staphylococcal infection but, as in this picture, there may be multiple superficial pustules suggestive of a herpetic origin.

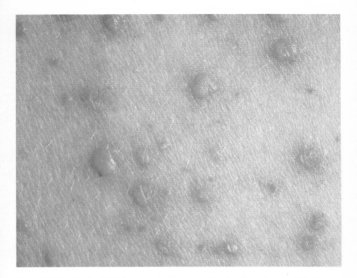

Fig. 50 Varicella (chicken pox). The eruption is discrete, each lesion starting as a macule which rapidly becomes papular and then vesicular. The eruption develops in crops and is denser on trunk and face than on the limbs. The lesions are very superficial and soon crust over or are scratched, so that vesicles may not easily be seen.

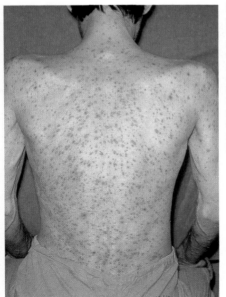

Fig. 51 Varicella. This general view of severe varicella shows the characteristic distribution with superficial lesions at different stages of development. The rash is most dense centrally, on the face and trunk, and grades off towards the periphery.

26

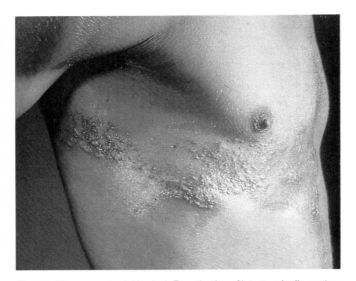

Fig. 52 Herpes zoster (shingles). Reactivation of latent varicella-zoster virus is heralded by pain in area of distribution of the affected nerve roots. The pain may accompany, or may precede by several days, the first signs of erythema, which is quickly followed by the development of a vesiculopustular eruption. By courtesy of Dr. J. F. John, Jr.

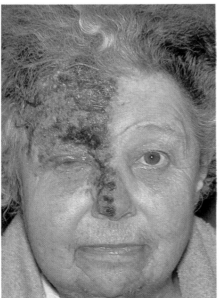

Fig. 53 Herpes zoster of the ophthalmic division of the trigeminal nerve. This is the division most commonly affected, although maxillary or mandibular herpes are occasionally seen. Lesions of the nose to the tip indicate that the naso-ciliary branch is involved and that the eye may be affected.

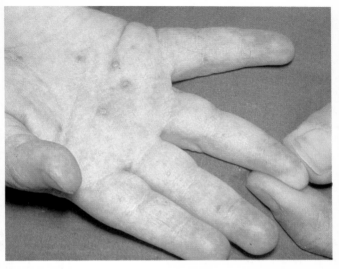

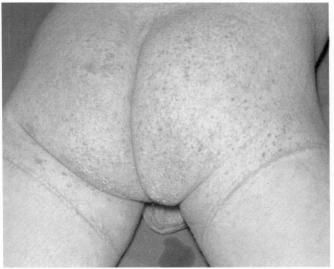

Fig. 54 Hand, foot and mouth disease. Enteroviral rashes are common and some types such as echoviruses 9, 16 and 4 and Coxsackie A9 and A16 are especially likely to cause rashes. Hand, foot and mouth disease is usually caused by Coxsackie A16. There are a few lax vesicles on the hands and feet; macules and vesicles are seen in the mouth. Some patients have a maculopapular rash on buttocks and thighs as seen in the lower photograph and sometimes this form of rash is seen alone without a vesicular element.

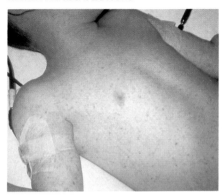

Fig. 55 Rocky Mountain spotted fever (*Rickettsia rickettsii*). The rash appears after several days of fever, starting peripherally and spreading centrally to the trunk. It is initially macular but later becomes petechial and purpuric. Sometimes large ecchymoses develop. By courtesy of Dr. T. F. Sellers, Jr.

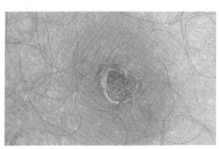

Fig. 56 East African tick typhus (*Rickettsia conorii*). The site of the initiating tick bite is often seen as an eschar in scrub typhus and in fièvre boutonneuse. Here, in the healing stage, there is a central scab and surrounding erythema.

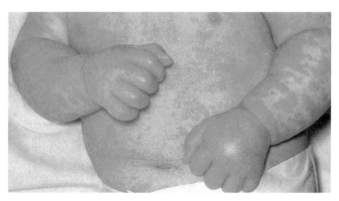

Fig. 57 Kawasaki disease. The aetiology is obscure but one hypothesis points to a hypersensitivity response to a rickettsial agent. Diagnosis is provisionally based on identifying at least five of the six main features: fever for at least five days not responding to antibiotics, dry, red oral mucosa, conjunctival congestion, red indurated oedema of the extremities and a polymorphic, mainly central rash. The last two features are shown here.

Cutaneous Manifestations of Bacterial Infection

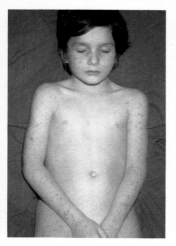 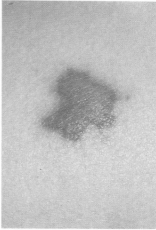

Fig. 58 Meningococcal septicaemia. The most common appearance is a mixed petechial and maculo papular rash more prevalent on the extremities and extensor surfaces. Anything from petechiae to large ecchymoses may be seen. The central part of an irregular ecchymosis like this may become purulent and then necrotic followed by ulceration and skin loss. The smaller lesions heal with scarring. In the most severe form, the Waterhouse-Friderichsen syndrome, the whole skin may become rapidly covered with purpura, within a few hours of onset.

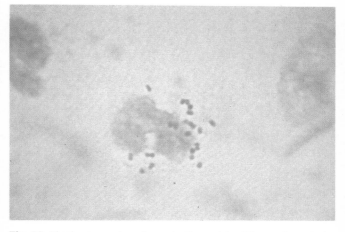

Fig. 59 Meningococcal septicaemia. Gram stain of the cerebrospinal fluid deposits showing intracellular Gram-negative diplococci. The organisms may also be found in scrapes from skin lesions. By courtesy of A. E. Prevost.

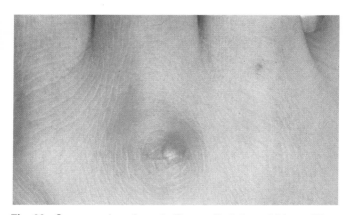

Fig. 60. Gonococcal septicaemia. The manifestations of this condition include skin lesions, arthritis, tenosynovitis and occasionally endocarditis. The skin lesions are often scanty. Pustules with surrounding purpura are the most common feature, but sometimes, as in this picture, the purpuric element is absent. Macules, papules, purpura and even areas of purpuric necrosis may also be present. Lesions are most often seen on the hands and feet. By courtesy of Dr. T. F. Sellers, Jr.

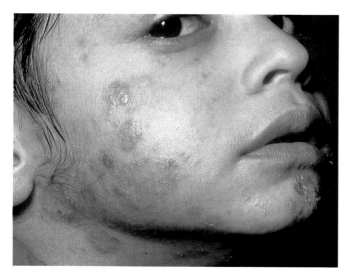

Fig. 61 Impetigo. This is a superficial infection caused by streptococci, staphylococci or a combination of both. Clusters of superficial vesicles rapidly become purulent and form yellow adherent crusts. New lesions develop at other sites and, if untreated, the lesions may slowly enlarge and multiply over weeks or months. This boy's face shows several affected areas, some of which have scabbed.

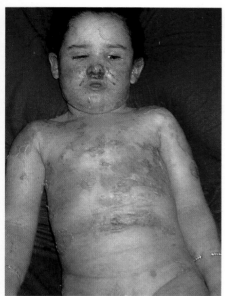

Fig. 62 Staphylococcal scalded skin syndrome (Lyell's syndrome). Some strains of staphylococci of phage group II produce an exfoliative toxin. Multiple superficial areas of skin loss are seen, with a strong resemblance to scalding. The impetiginous lesion at the root of the nose was the original site of staphylococcal infection. The lesions soon regress after starting treatment with flucloxacillin given orally.

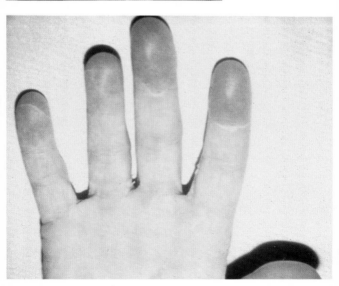

Fig. 63 Toxic shock syndrome. Many of the manifestations of this disease (fever, hypotension, generalized erythematous rash, nausea and vomiting, diarrhoea) are non-specific, but the characteristic desquamation, which commonly involves the hands and feet, is rarely seen in other conditions. By courtesy of Dr. R. T. Ball.

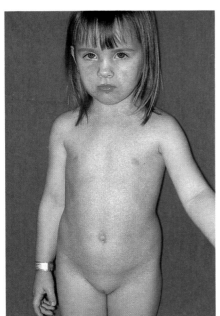

Fig. 64 Scarlet fever. The rash begins as a facial erythema sparing the area round the mouth, and spreads to the trunk and limbs. The classical appearance is described as a punctate erythema, and is followed by extensive peeling which may continue for two or three weeks. The tongue, furred at first, later looks raw with prominent papillae.

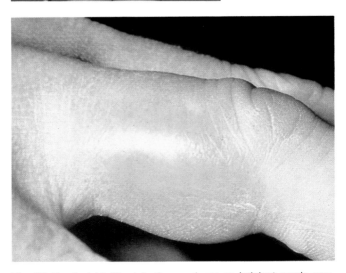

Fig. 65 Erysipeloid. The infection produces an indolent purple non-purulent swelling at the site of infection. It is an occupational disease of fish and meat handlers as the organism (*Erysipelothrix rhusiopathiae*) is found in many wild and domestic animals. The finger is a common site of infection.

33

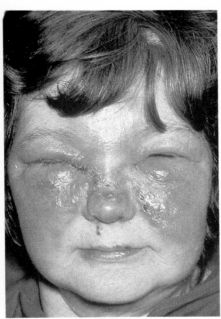

Fig. 66 Erysipelas, caused by *Streptococcus pyogenes*. The raised red indurated area of inflammation has spread rapidly to give a butterfly distribution with blistering on the affected areas. The eyes are closed by oedema, but are unaffected.

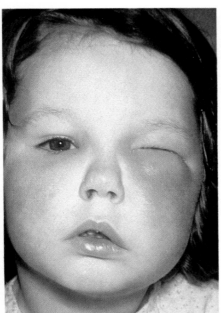

Fig. 67 Orbital cellulitis. Erysipelas is usually streptococcal but other forms of cellulitis may be streptococcal or staphylococcal. Orbital cellulitis, as seen in this child, may be associated with underlying maxillary sinusitis. *Haemophilus influenzae* group B causes an unusual form of cellulitis with a purple bruised appearance usually seen on the cheek.

34

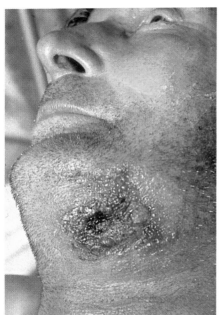

Fig. 68 Anthrax. In the Western World this is a rare occupational disease associated with contact with imported hides, wool and hair. The cutaneous form begins as a small papule and is soon surrounded by vesicles. The central area ulcerates and dries to form a black eschar. There is much surrounding oedema. Later the eschar spreads to cover the previously vesicular area. By courtesy of Dr. F. J. Nye.

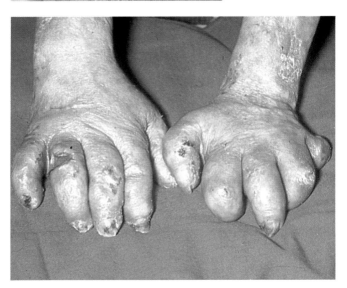

Fig. 69 Leprosy (Hansen's disease). The neuropathy of lepromatous leprosy leads to ulceration, loss of tissue and eventually to gross deformity. Acid-fast bacilli are seen in skin snips or biopsies.

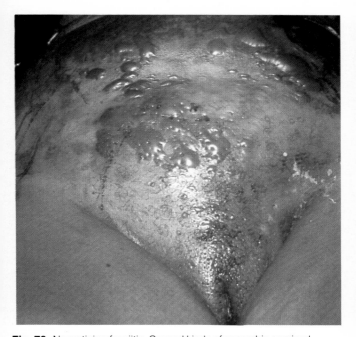

Fig. 70 Necrotizing fasciitis. Several kinds of anaerobic or mixed infections of skin and subcutaneous tissues are seen, especially in patients with diabetes or those who are generally ill. Ischaemic tissues are vulnerable. Multiple bullae and areas of necrosis are seen in the abdominal wall. The organisms isolated were all anaerobes, consisting of peptostreptococci, *Bacteroides fragilis* and *Bacteroides melaninogenicus*. By courtesy of Dr. W. M. Rambo.

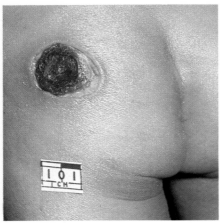

Fig. 71 Ecthyma gangrenosum. This type of lesion is seen in two clinical settings, in this case in an immunodeficient child who developed *Pseudomonas septicaemia*. A similar lesion is found as one of the dermal manifestations of ulcerative colitis. Sometimes the edge is raised and the lesion can be mistaken for a cutaneous mycosis such as blastomycosis or sporotrichosis.

Cutaneous Manifestations of Infection:
Fungal and Other Miscellaneous Infections

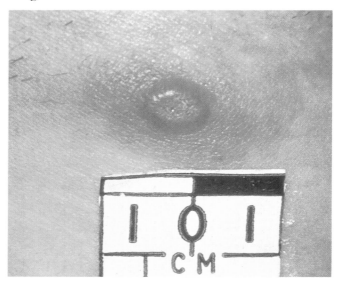

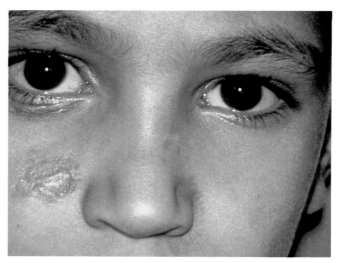

Fig. 72 Cutaneous leishmaniasis. This shows an early stage of infection with *Leishmania donovani*. After an incubation period of several months, an itchy papule with surrounding erythema develops at the site of a sandfly bite. A shallow ulcer develops, slowly enlarges and later heals leaving the characteristic puckered scar.

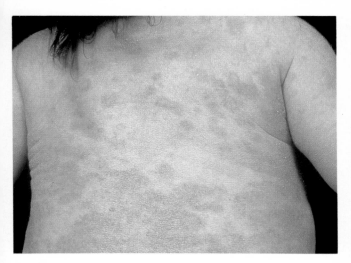

Fig. 73 Generalized cutaneous candidiasis. This can be seen even in patients without immunodeficiency, especially in infants as a complication of a napkin rash. Irregular, slightly raised red or brownish-red patches of ranging size give a characteristic appearance, as seen in this baby. By courtesy of the Institute of Dermatology.

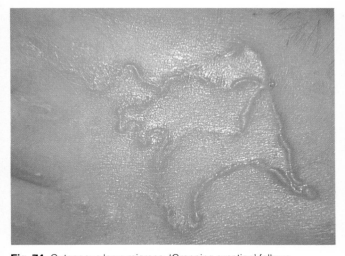

Fig. 74 Cutaneous larva migrans. 'Creeping eruption' follows infestation with larval nematodes of various species, usually dog or cat hookworms. A serpiginous raised lesion appears which can spread rapidly, disappear or appear at multiple sites. The lesions are intensely itchy. Treatment with local or systemic thiabendazole is usually effective. By courtesy of Dr. K. A. Riley.

38

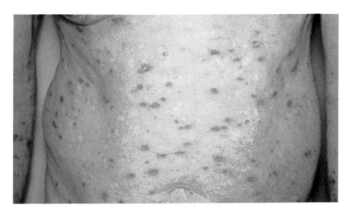

Fig. 75 Pediculosis. Of the three forms of louse infestation, head lice are seen least frequently. Their presence is indicated by nits attached to the scalp hair. Pubic lice ('crabs') can often be seen as well as nits and bite marks, while body lice are seen only on clothing. Vagabond's disease, seen in this photograph, is a result of heavy infestation and poor hygiene; there is a generalized rash with secondary pigmentation and lichenified skin. By courtesy of Dr. S. Olansky.

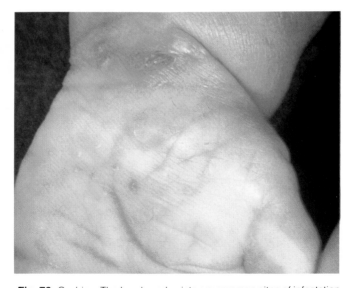

Fig. 76 Scabies. The hands and wrists are common sites of infestation with *Sarcoptes scabiei*. The rash is often complicated by secondary infection, by the effects of scratching and by allergic reactions. Although the rash is often most prominent on other parts of the body – although not on the head and neck – mites can usually be found only on the hands and wrists, in the short linear burrows.

Infections of the Gastrointestinal Tract and Biliary System

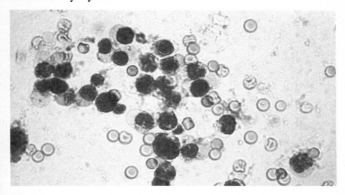

Fig. 77 Shigellosis. In bacterial diseases due to invasive microorganisms, inflammatory cells and red blood cells are usually present in the faeces. These may be visualized by mixing a fleck of mucus with a drop of methylene blue stain and examining the preparation under a glass cover slip. By courtesy of Dr. H. L. DuPont.

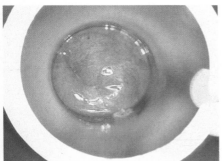

Fig. 78 Shigellosis. In mild cases, sigmoidoscopic examination may reveal only diffuse hyperaemia of the colonic mucosa and a thin whitish exudate which is made up of fibrin and polymorphonuclear leucocytes. By courtesy of Dr. R. H. Gilman.

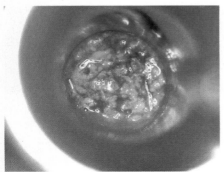

Fig. 79 Shigellosis. Severe cases may develop an extensive pseudomembranous colitis, as in this fatal case due to *Shigella dysenteriae* type 1. By courtesy of Drs. R. H. Gilman and F. Koster.

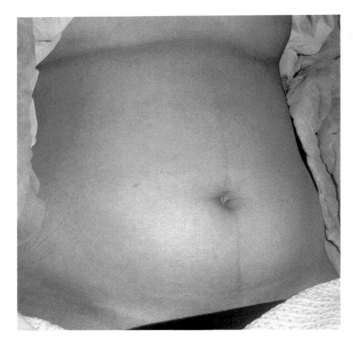

Fig. 80 Typhoid fever. Rose spots are small (2-4 mm) erythematous maculopapular lesions which blanch on pressure. They characteristically appear in small numbers (less than a dozen) on the abdomen and disappear within a few hours or days. By courtesy of Dr. G. D. W. McKendrick.

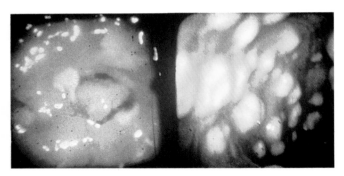

Fig. 81 Antibiotic-associated colitis. The characteristic lesions, seen on sigmoidoscopic examination in approximately half the patients, are whitish or yellowish plaques, which may be surrounded by haemorrhagic borders. Other patients exhibit only diffuse inflammatory changes. The disease is caused by a cytotoxin produced by *Clostridium difficile*. By courtesy of Dr. F. Pittman (left), Dr. R. Fekety (right).

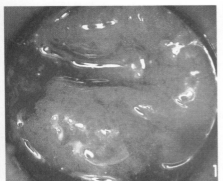

Fig. 82 Amoebic colitis. This is a world-wide disease caused by invasion of the bowel wall by the protozoan parasite *Entamoeba histolytica*. In most patients sigmoidoscopic examination reveals only diffuse inflammation of the colon, without ulceration. By courtesy of Dr. R. H. Gilman.

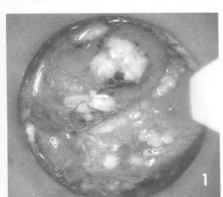

Fig. 83 Amoebic colitis. More severe cases show the 'textbook' lesions: deep ulcers with overlying purulent exudate. By courtesy of Dr. R. H. Gilman.

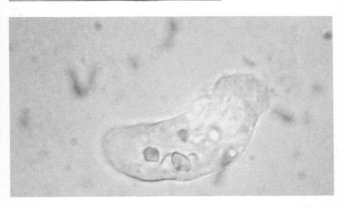

Fig. 84 Amoebic colitis. Motile trophozoites, often containing red blood cells, may be seen in a wet mount of material obtained via the sigmoidoscope from an area of purulent exudate. By courtesy of Dr. H. L. DuPont.

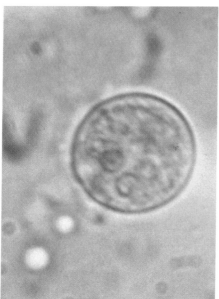

Fig. 85 Amoebic colitis. Non-diarrhoeal stools often contain only cysts, which are round, with a refractile cell wall and multiple (usually four) nuclei. By courtesy of Dr. H. L. DuPont.

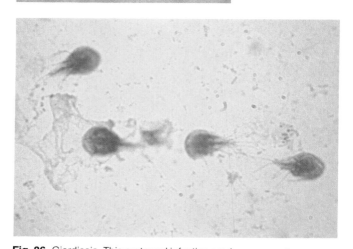

Fig. 86 Giardiasis. This protozoal infection produces an acute diarrhoea which may become chronic; sometimes there is malabsorption and even frank steatorrhoea. If three stool examinations have been negative for *Giardia lamblia* in a patient suspected of having giardiasis, trophozoites can be looked for in mucus stripped from an Enterotest string pulled from the duodenum after overnight passage. Note the characteristic shape, paired nuclei and multiple flagella. By courtesy of Dr. F. Pittman.

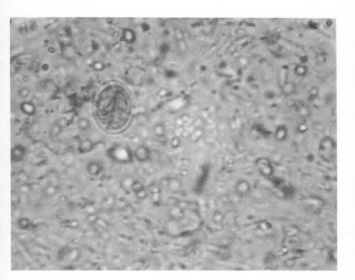

Fig. 87 Giardiasis. Cysts of *Giardia lamblia* are ovoid in shape, with a prominent cyst wall, granular cytoplasm, and at least two nuclei. By courtesy of Dr. H. L. DuPont.

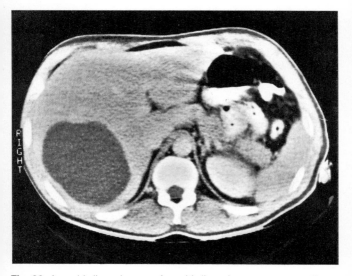

Fig. 88 Amoebic liver abscess. Amoebic liver abscesses are usually single and located in the right lobe, and may be extremely large. Computerized tomographic (CT) scanning, as shown here, and radionuclide scanning are valuable techniques for the detection and localization of intrahepatic abscesses. By courtesy of Dr. F. Pittman.

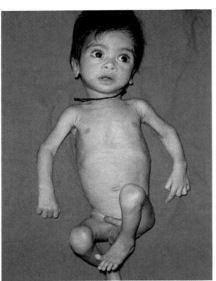

Fig. 89 Infantile gastroenteritis. This dehydrated and malnourished baby exemplifies the problem of gastroenteritis as a global cause of serious morbidity in infancy and childhood. There are numerous causal agents. In most countries rotaviruses are the most frequent, especially in the winter months. Enterotoxigenic and enteropathogenic *Escherichia coli* are also important, but in many such illnesses, a causal organism cannot yet be identified.

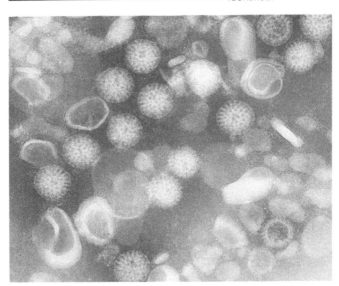

Fig. 90 Viral gastroenteritis. Of the known infectious causes of diarrhoea in children, the most important are the rotaviruses, so-called because of the 'spoked-wheel' appearance of the viral particles (about 70 nm in diameter). Rotaviruses are usually present in such large amounts in diarrhoeal stools that they can be identified directly by electron microscopy. By courtesy of Prof. C. R. Madeley.

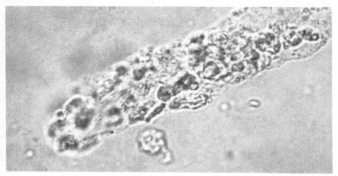

Fig. 91 Acute pyelonephritis. A useful sign in bacterial infection of the kidney is the presence of casts containing white blood cells in the urinary sediment. This high power view of urine sediment shows a tubular cast containing many white blood cells in various stages of degeneration. Failure to observe white cell casts does not rule out the presence of renal involvement in urinary tract infection. By courtesy of Dr. S. Rous.

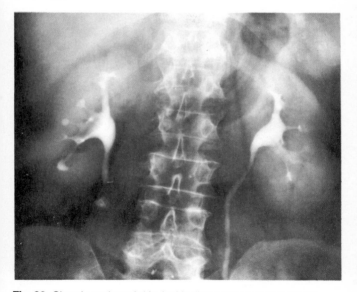

Fig. 92 Chronic pyelonephritis. In this disease there is asymmetric contraction and distortion of the kidney, with deep cortical scars overlying dilated and blunted calices. In this intravenous pyelogram the apposition of cortical scarring and distortion of the caliceal system is easily seen in the right kidney, whereas the left kidney appears normal. By courtesy of Dr. C. N. Griffin.

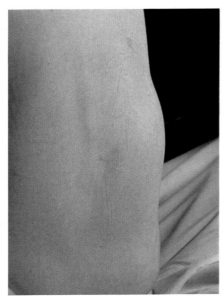

Fig. 93 Perinephric abscess. Renal infection may extend through the capsule of the kidney to produce an abscess in the perinephric space. The patient may have fever with few local signs or may have evidence of pyelonephritis and a bulging mass in the flank. By courtesy of Dr. P. Hohl.

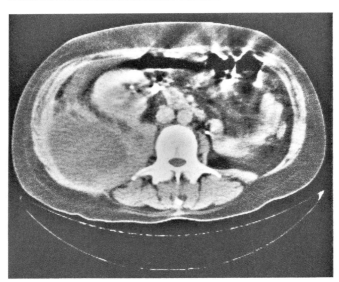

Fig. 94 Perinephric abscess. Computerized tomographic (CT) scanning and ultrasound studies have greatly aided in the diagnosis of this condition. This CT scan shows a large abscess in the right perinephric space, with marked anterior displacement of the right kidney. By courtesy of Dr. P. Hohl.

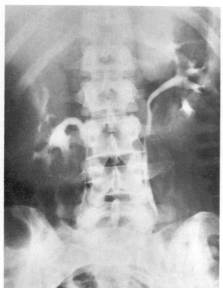

Fig. 95 Renal carbuncle. In haematogenic pyelonephritis, usually from *Staphylococcus aureus,* or in ascending infection due to *Escherichia coli,* a large intrarenal abscess may form. This intravenous urogram shows a hyperlucent mass in the upper pole of the right kidney, with distortion of the upper lobe calices. By courtesy of Dr. C. N. Griffin.

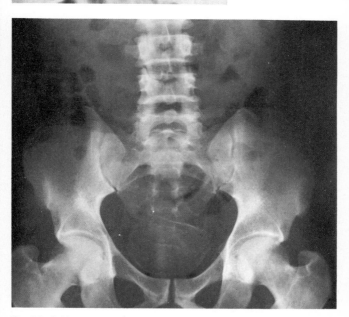

Fig. 96 Schistosomiasis. A late stage in the chronic granulomatous reaction due to *Schistosoma haematobium* infection is calcification outlining the bladder wall, as shown in this plain abdominal X-ray.

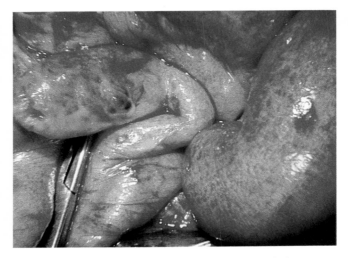

Fig. 97 Acute apendicitis. This operating room photograph shows a grossly inflamed appendix and an area of necrosis where perforation has occurred at the site of a faecalith. The adjacent serosal surface shows congestion and fibrinous exudate. By courtesy of Dr. M. Anderson.

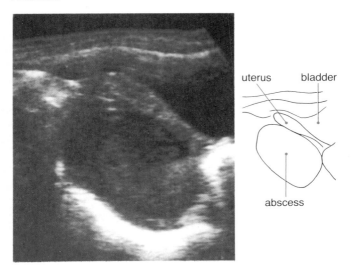

Fig. 98 Appendiceal abscess. Perforation may be followed by generalized peritonitis or the infection may become localized as an appendiceal abscess. This ultrasound study shows an abscess in the pouch of Douglas secondary to a ruptured appendix (lateral view). By courtesy of Dr. A. E. A. Joseph.

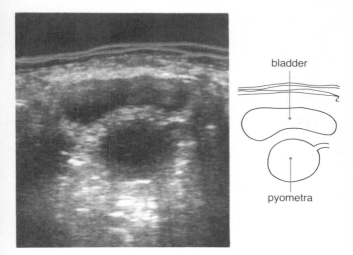

bladder

pyometra

Fig. 99 Pelvic inflammatory disease. This term covers a wide variety of conditions, often of uncertain aetiology. The gonococcus is a common cause, and chlamydia is being increasingly recognized in cases of PID. *Bacteroides* species and other anaerobes, with or without facultative bacteria like *Escherichia coli* are often found when abscesses develop. This ultrasound study shows a large pyometra. By courtesy of Dr. A. E. A. Joseph.

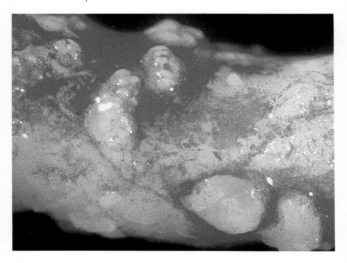

Fig. 100 Pelvic actinomycosis. This infection may be increasing in frequency because of an association with intrauterine contraceptive devices. This picture shows part of an IUD studded with 'molar-tooth' colonies of *Actinomyces israelii*. By courtesy of A. E. Prevost.

Disseminated Infections

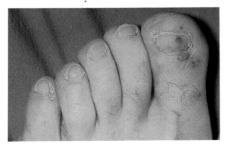

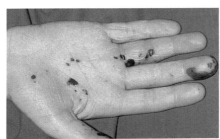

Fig. 101 Bacterial endocarditis. Widespread skin lesions may sometimes be seen, especially in acute staphylococcal endocarditis. This patient showed numerous ecchymoses of his hands and feet during the course of staphylococcal septicaemia, and signs of aortic valve involvement soon appeared.

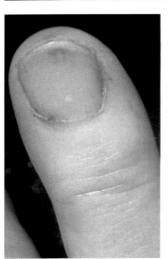

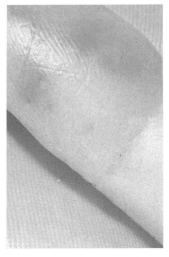

Fig. 102 Two diagnostically important peripheral manifestations of infective endocarditis are splinter haemorrhages (left) and Osler's nodes (right). These painful erythematous nodular lesions may be due to deposition of immune complexes in blood vessel walls, but bacteria have been cultured from them in a few instances, suggesting that they may be embolic in nature. By courtesy of Dr. J. F. John, Jr.

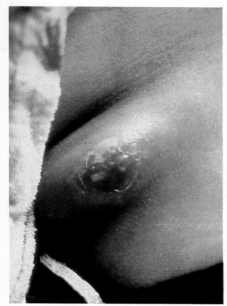

Fig. 103 Plague. In bubonic plague, the most common form of infection in humans by *Yersinia pestis*, the organisms multiply rapidly at the site of the bite of an infected flea, and spread to the regional lymph nodes, producing the characteristic suppurative lymphadenitis (bubo). This patient exhibits an advanced stage of inguinal lymphadenitis, in which the lymph nodes have undergone suppuration and the lesion has drained spontaneously. By courtesy of Dr. J. R. Cantey.

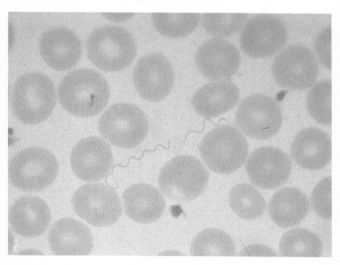

Fig. 104 Relapsing fever. This may be either an epidemic louse-borne human disease caused by *Borrelia recurrentis* or a tick-borne zoonosis caused by various species of *Borrelia*. During the febrile phase the organisms are present in the blood, either as tightly-coiled helical spirochaetes, as shown here, or as loosely-coiled forms. By courtesy of Dr. T. F. Sellers, Jr.

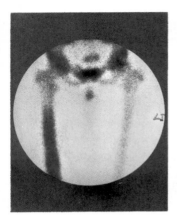
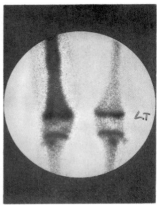

Fig. 105 Osteomyelitis. In the early stages of bacterial infection of bone (the first 10-14 days, before extensive destruction of bone has taken place), X-rays may not reveal the characteristic changes of bone destruction, periosteal reaction and sequestrum formation. Radionuclide scanning with isotopes of technetium and gallium may be positive as early as three days after the onset of symptoms, before extensive lysis of bone has occurred. This technetium 99 methylene diphosphonate scan shows markedly increased uptake in the lower two-thirds of the right femur. By courtesy of Dr. D. Ackery.

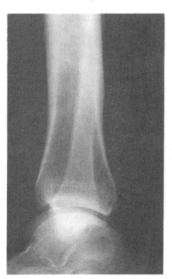
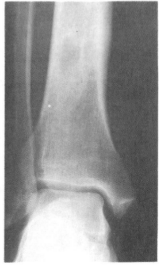

Fig. 106 Osteomyelitis. This patient exhibits a fully developed Brodie's abscess of the tibia, with surrounding sclerosis of bone and elevation of the periosteum. By courtesy of Dr. D. Ackery.

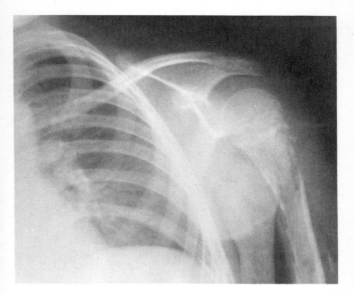

Fig. 107 Osteomyelitis. This radiograph shows far-advanced osteomyelitis of the humerus in a child, with irregular destruction of bone and a great deal of periosteal reaction.

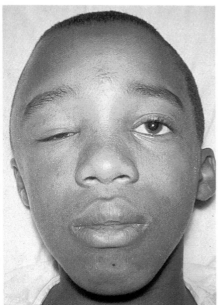

Fig. 108 Acute osteomyelitis. Osteomyelitis may develop secondary to a contiguous focus of infection, often related to surgical procedure or trauma. This case of osteomyelitis of the right frontal bone due to *Staphylococcus aureus* was associated with infection of the right frontal sinus ('Pott's puffy tumour'). By courtesy of Dr. T. F. Sellers, Jr.

54

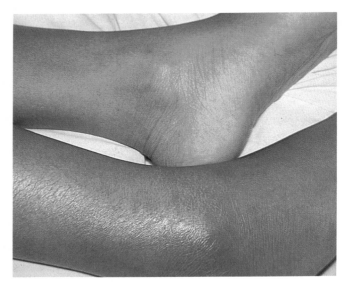

Fig. 109 Gonococcal arthritis. Patients with bacteraemia due to *Neisseria gonorrhoeae* may have marked systemic symptoms with fever, polyarthralgia, tenosynovitis, and characteristic skin lesions, or may present with a monarticular septic arthritis. This 24-year old woman has septic arthritis of the right ankle with marked erythema and swelling of the ankle and leg. By courtesy of Dr. T. F. Sellers, Jr.

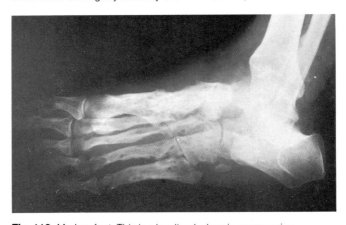

Fig. 110 Madura foot. This is a localized, chronic, progressive destructive infection involving the skin, subcutaneous tissues, muscle, and bone. It is caused by soil organisms, including a number of different species of fungi. The granulomatous process gradually destroys the architecture of the involved bones and soft tissues, with production of deep abscesses and multiple draining fistulous tracts.

Infections and the Eye

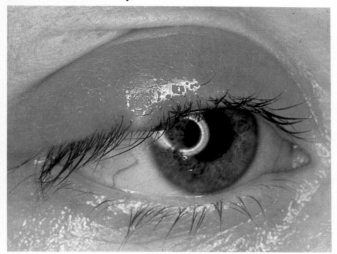

Fig. 111 Stye or hordeolum. This is a localized infection of the eyelid, usually caused by *Staphylococcus aureus*. This patient has generalized swelling and redness of the upper lid with a localized collection of pus near the lid margin. By courtesy of Mr. R. J. Marsh and Ms. Sue Ford.

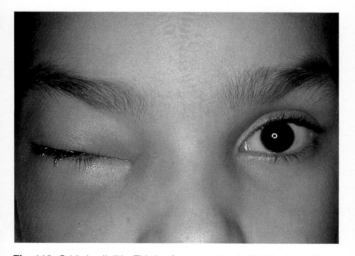

Fig. 112 Orbital cellulitis. This is often associated with infection of the adjacent paranasal sinuses and is usually of streptococcal or staphylococcal aetiology. The main features are fever, pain in the orbit, tenderness, swelling and erythema of the lids. By courtesy of Mr. R. J. Marsh and Ms. Sue Ford.

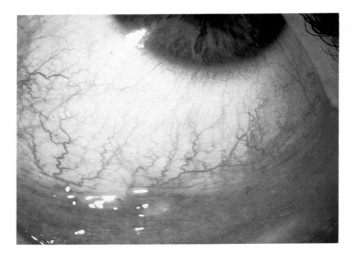

Fig. 113 Acute conjunctivitis. Acute infection of the conjunctiva may be caused by viruses, bacteria, or chlamydia. All forms of conjunctivitis are accompanied by itching, excessive lacrimation and more or less severe conjunctival injection. Typically the degree of hyperaemia diminishes in severity towards the cornea; in iritis the hyperaemia is greatest at the limbus. By courtesy of Mr. R. J. Marsh and Ms. Sue Ford.

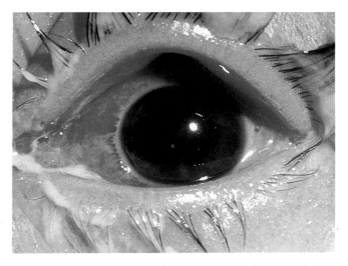

Fig. 114 Purulent conjunctivitis. In bacterial conjunctivitis a purulent discharge is typically present, as in this patient. The bacteria most commonly involved are *Streptococcus pneumoniae, Staphylococcus aureus,* and *Haemophilus influenzae.* By courtesy of Dr. M. Tapert.

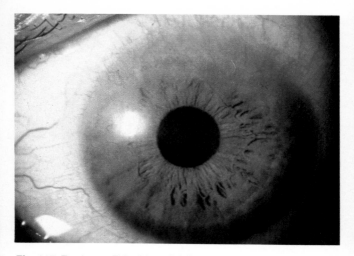

Fig. 115 Trachoma. This chlamydial disease is a major cause of blindness, especially in less developed areas of the world. An initial follicular conjunctivitis and keratitis is followed by development of trachomatous pannus, at first in the upper half of the corneal margin and then spreading over the cornea. Note new vessel formation and hazy upper corneal margin. By courtesy of Mr. R. J. Marsh and Ms. Sue Ford.

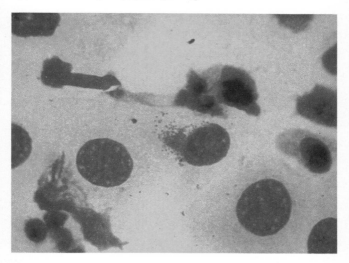

Fig. 116 Inclusion conjunctivitis. This infection, which is also caused by *Chlamydia trachomatis,* may occur from infancy through adulthood. The organism may be identified in conjunctival scrapings, stained with Giemsa stain, as an intracytoplasmic basophilic inclusion consisting of numerous small uniform particles. By courtesy of Dr. S. Fisher-Hoch.

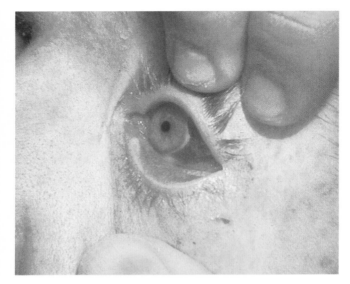

Fig. 117 Leptospirosis. Acute conjunctivitis and conjunctival haemorrhages are often seen in leptospirosis. Uveitis is seen in only about 2% of patients. By courtesy of Dr. T. F. Sellers, Jr.

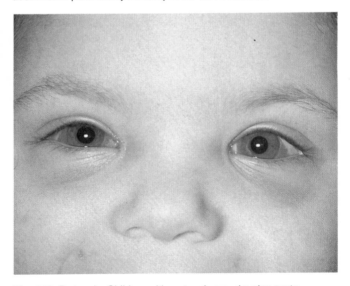

Fig. 118 Pertussis. Children with pertussis may develop acute subconjunctival haemorrhages after a prolonged bout of coughing. These haemorrhages are naturally alarming to the parents but clear quickly without complications.

59

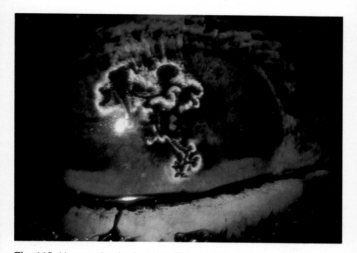

Fig. 119 Herpes simplex keratitis. The most important viral cause of keratitis is herpes simplex. The lesion usually begins as a punctate keratitis which may have an obstinately recurrent course. In the more severe forms ulcers appear, either as a large ulcer with an irregular edge, or in the pathognomonic dendritic shape, seen here after staining with fluorescein.

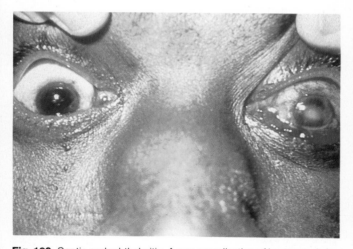

Fig. 120 Septic endophthalmitis. A rare complication of bacteraemia is septic endophthalmitis usually due to *Streptococcus pneumoniae, Neisseria meningitidis* or *Staphylococcus aureus*. In this patient the endophthalmitis accompanied pneumococcal bacteraemia. There is general hyperaemia of the eye, and pus in the anterior chamber can be seen as a white opacity. Hypopyon is also present. By courtesy of Dr. T. F. Sellers, Jr.

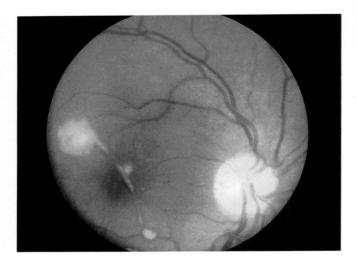

Fig. 121 *Candida* endophthalmitis. Dots and blobs of white fluffy exudate, located in the vitreous just anterior to the retina, may be the only clues to the presence of systemic candidiasis. By courtesy of Dr. P. Hohl.

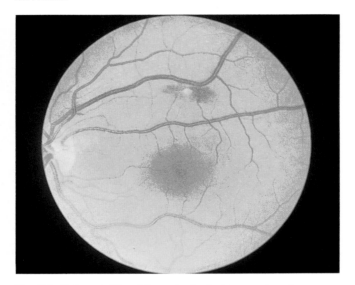

Fig. 122 Roth spot. This white-centred retinal haemorrhage is an important diagnostic sign of metastatic infection, most commonly seen in infective endocarditis. It is, however, occasionally seen in non-infectious conditions such as systemic lupus erythematosus and leukaemia.

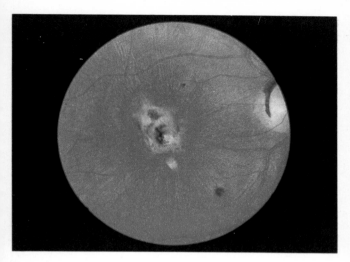

Fig. 123 Histoplasmosis. Ocular involvement in histoplasmosis is usually manifested by a multifocal peripheral chorioretinitis which heals to form yellowish, well-defined scars. Macular involvement, with significant loss of visual acuity, is unfortunately common. Characteristically there are no inflammatory signs in the vitreous or aqueous. By courtesy of Dr. T. F. Sellers, Jr.

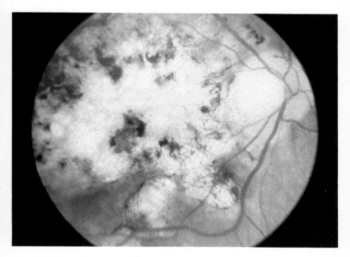

Fig. 124 Toxoplasmosis. Ocular toxoplasmosis is usually the result of congenital infection, sometimes with episodes of reactivation during childhood or adulthood. The lesion is a focal destructive chorioretinitis which leaves well-defined, heavily-pigmented scars, especially in the macular region.

62

Tuberculosis

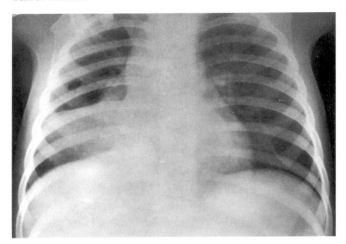

Fig. 125 Tuberculosis. Primary infection is usually a clinically silent event, marked only by a positive tuberculin reaction. The radiological features of primary pulmonary infection are a peripheral shadow of the primary focus, enlarged hilar nodes, or, more commonly, an area of consolidation, as here, affecting the right middle lobe.

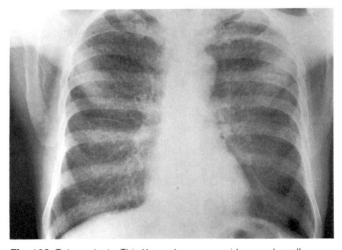

Fig. 126 Tuberculosis. This X-ray shows very widespread small discrete shadows in both lung fields. The patient had miliary tuberculosis, a sequel of haematogenous dissemination of the organism which may develop in the post-primary phase or in patients with long-standing latent infection. Miliary tuberculosis is also encountered in patients with immunosuppression.

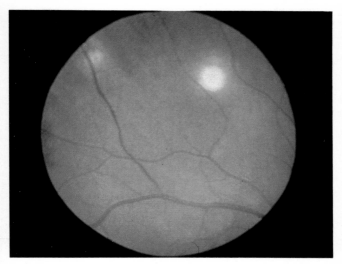

Fig. 127 Tuberculosis. The diagnosis of miliary tuberculosis can usually be made by a combination of evidence from contact history, chest radiograph, tuberculin testing and sometimes liver biopsy. Some patients with miliary disease also have tuberculous meningitis. Tubercles can occasionally be seen directly, in the choroid, as seen in this photograph. At an earlier stage the lesions are pinker and less well-defined. By courtesy of Dr. J. A. Innes.

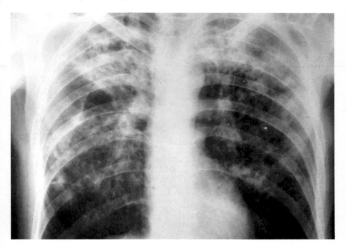

Fig. 128 Tuberculosis. This radiograph is typical of advanced chronic pulmonary disease. There is extensive nodular shadowing in both lungs, especially in the upper zones. Both upper lobes are contracted and there is cavitation in the right upper lobe.

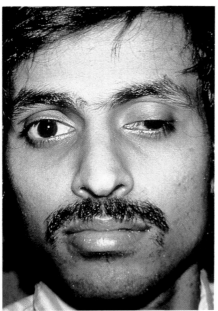

Fig. 129
Tuberculosis. The changes of tuberculous meningitis are most marked at the base of the brain. Of the many possible complications, cranial nerve palsies are among the commonest. This patient was making satisfactory general progress when he developed a left oculomotor palsy, shown by the ptosis and lateral deviation of the left eye caused by unopposed action of the lateral rectus.

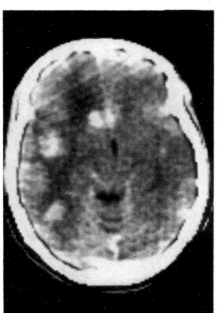

Fig. 130
Tuberculosis. These multiple rounded lesions with surrounding oedema, shown on the CT scan, are tuberculomas. Similar appearances may be seen in pyogenic abscess, fungal lesions, and meningiomas. By courtesy of Dr. J. Ambrose.

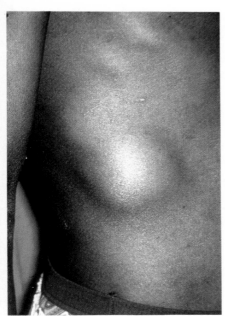

Fig. 131
Tuberculosis. Bones and joints may be affected by tuberculosis at any time in the natural history of the infection, from less than a year to many decades after primary infection. There may be adjacent caseation and bone disease may present as a cold abscess, as in this patient with an indolent swelling of the chest wall. Radiographs showed tuberculosis of the underlying ribs.

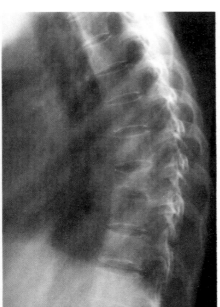

Fig. 132
Tuberculosis. Symptoms of bone tuberculosis may long precede radiographic abnormalities, although isotope bone scanning provides a more sensitive method for the detection of single or multiple tuberculous foci. This lateral spinal radiograph of a young Asian patient with backache shows compression and loss of a vertebral body with erosion of the anterior edge.

66

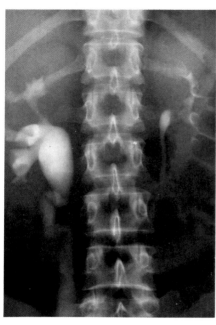

Fig. 133
Tuberculosis. Genito-
urinary tuberculosis
often develops in older
patients in whom
infection has long
been latent. This
intravenous urogram
shows irregularity of
the calices with
caliceal abscesses in
the upper pole of the
right kidney, and a
dilated ureter. The left
kidney is normal.

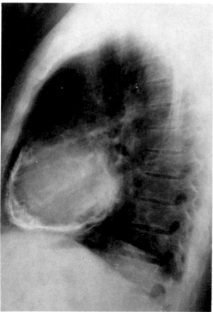

Fig. 134
Tuberculosis.
Pericarditis caused by
tuberculous infection
is a rare disease in the
Western World, but is
quite common in some
parts of Africa. It may
be detected at the
acute stage and
features of tamponade
may develop then or
much later, when the
radiographic
appearances of
pericardial calcification
may be seen.

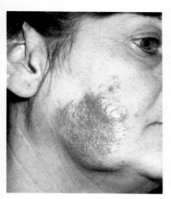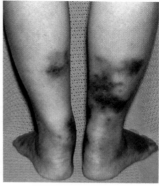

Fig. 135 Tuberculosis. Skin manifestations of tuberculosis are uncommon. Lupus vulgaris may develop in previously normal skin or at the site of a tuberculous sinus. A red-brown plaque of indurated tissue spreads slowly with eventual scarring and tissue destruction (left). Carcinoma may develop as a late complication. Another type of skin involvement in tuberculosis is seen in the various forms of tuberculide; in one of these, Bazin's disease or erythema induratum, dark, lumpy, indurated lesions develop on the legs and may form indolent ragged ulcers (right). The patients show a high degree of tuberculin sensitivity and the lesions respond to antituberculous chemotherapy.

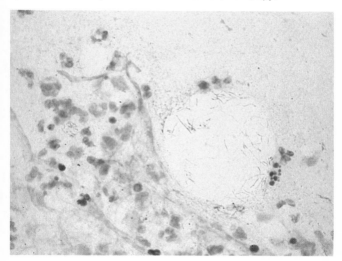

Fig. 136 Tuberculosis. Mycobacterium tuberculosis can be seen in sputum as delicate bacilli of various length, staining pink in the Ziehl-Neelsen stain. They can also be seen by fluorescence miscroscopy. Infectivity is closely related to the presence of tubercule bacilli on direct examination of the sputum. By courtesy of Dr. J. F. John, Jr.

Parasitic Infections

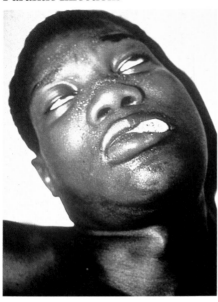

Fig. 137 African trypanosomiasis. In both forms of African trypanosomiasis (sleeping sickness), the West African due to *Trypanosoma brucei gambiense* and the East African due to *T. b. rhodesiense,* a meningoencephalitis results and causes much of the morbidity and mortality of this disease. In both forms, the final stage of the encephalitis is a profound stupor. By courtesy of Drs. M. E. Krampitz and P. de Raadt.

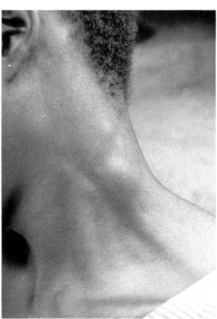

Fig. 138 African trypanosomiasis. During the acute phase of the illness organisms are found in the blood and lymph nodes, and a helpful diagnostic sign is enlargement of nodes in the posterior cervical triangle (Winterbottom's sign). By courtesy of Prof. P. G. Janssens.

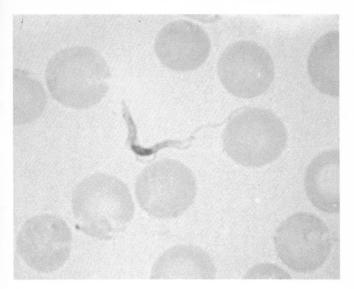

Fig. 139 African trypanosomiasis. *Trypanosoma brucei gambiense* in a thin blood smear from a patient from West Africa. Note the free flagellum and undulating membrane.

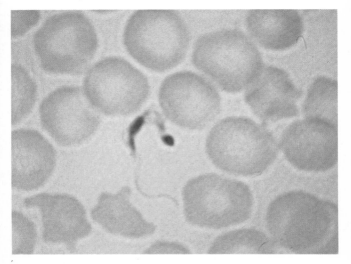

Fig. 140 American trypanosomiasis (Chagas' disease). Slender trypanosome form of *Trypanosoma cruzi* in a thin blood smear. Note prominent posterior kinetoplast and flagellum with elongated central nucleus. Giemsa stain. By courtesy of the Dept. of Medical Protozoology, London School of Hygiene and Tropical Medicine.

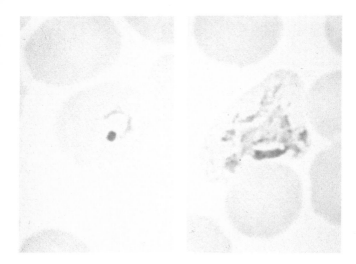

Fig. 141 Malaria. Thin blood smear showing (left) early trophozoite (ring form) and (right) a more mature amoeboid trophozoite of *Plasmodium vivax*. In malaria due to *P. vivax, P. malariae,* and *P. ovale,* early and late stages of the asexual forms are seen in erythrocytes. By courtesy of Dr. J. Parker-Williams.

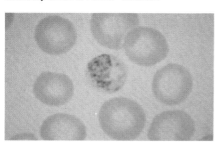

Fig. 142 Malaria. Thin blood smear showing mature trophozoite of *P. malariae.* Giemsa stain. By courtesy of Dr. J. Parker-Williams.

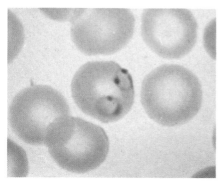

Fig. 143 Malaria. In malaria due to *Plasmodium falciparum,* early trophozoites (ring forms), shown here, greatly predominate over the more mature stages. Note two parasites within one red cell and double chromatin knobs. Giemsa stain. By courtesy of Dr. J. Parker-Williams.

71

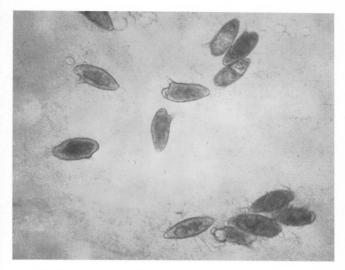

Fig. 144 Schistosomiasis. Worldwide, more than 200 million people are infected with one of the three species of human blood flukes belonging to the genus *Schistosoma.* Eggs of *S. mansoni,* shown here, have a characteristic lateral spine.

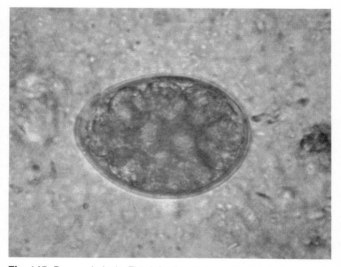

Fig. 145 Paragonimiasis. This infection is due to the lung fluke *Paragonimus westermani,* which is widely distributed in West Africa, India, the Far East and parts of Central and South America. Diagnosis depends upon finding the eggs in sputum or faeces. By courtesy of Dr. T. W. Holbrook.

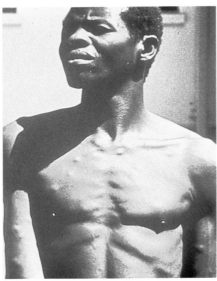

Fig. 146 Taeniasis (tapeworm infection). In man, infection with *Taenia solium* may produce either of two types of infection; gastrointestinal infection due to development of the adult worm in the gut, or systemic disease (cysticercosis) due to presence of larval cysts in various locations in the body. This patient has multiple subcutaneous cystic lesions containing the larvae, which are known as *Cysticercus cellulosae*. By courtesy of Dr. M. G. Schultz.

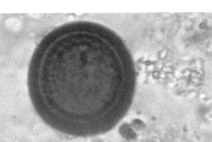

Fig. 147 Taeniasis. Egg of either *T. solium* or *T. saginata* in faeces containing hexacanth larva. By courtesy of Dr. T. W. Holbrook.

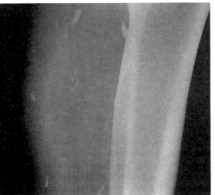

Fig. 148 Taeniasis. Radiograph of leg showing characteristic elongated calcified cysts of *T. solium*. At this site they produce no symptoms. When they occur in the brain they result in seizures or evidence of intracranial mass lesions.

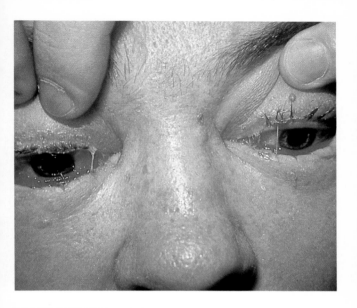

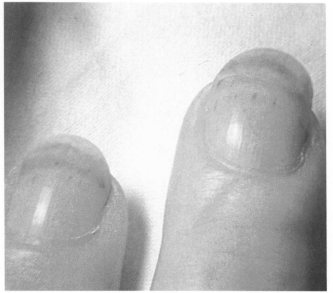

Fig. 149 Trichinosis. This disease is characterized by fever, muscle pain, periorbital oedema and eosinophilia. Occasionally severe conjunctivitis with conjunctival haemorrhages and splinter haemorrhages in the nail beds are seen. Courtesy of Dr. T. F. Sellers, Jr.

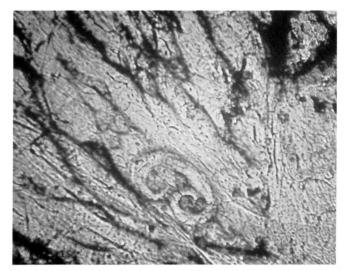

Fig. 150 Trichinosis. Once the diagnosis is suspected, it can be confirmed by finding the coiled larvae in a fresh specimen of muscle pressed between two glass slides. By courtesy of Dr. T. F. Sellers, Jr.

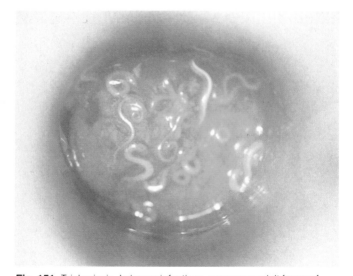

Fig. 151 Trichuriasis. In heavy infections, numerous adult forms of *Trichuris trichiura* may be seen on proctoscopic examination, as in this Malaysian child. The thin anterior 'whip' end of the worm is secured in the intestinal mucosa, and the thicker posterior end is seen within the lumen. By courtesy of Dr. R. H. Gilman.

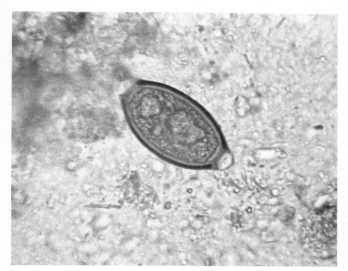

Fig. 152 Trichuriasis. Diagnosis is made by finding the characteristic eggs, which are barrel-shaped with a thick shell and translucent polar prominence, in the faeces.

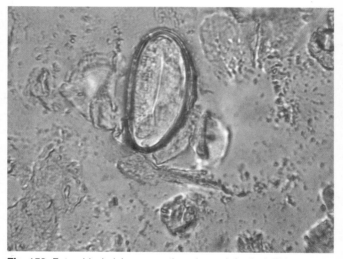

Fig. 153 Enterobiasis (pinworm or threadworm infection). This infection usually causes perianal itching, which may interfere with sleep. Diagnosis is made by finding the worm on the perianal region by flashlight at night, or more easily by pressing a strip of adhesive cellophane against the perianal region early in the morning and visualizing the characteristic eggs.

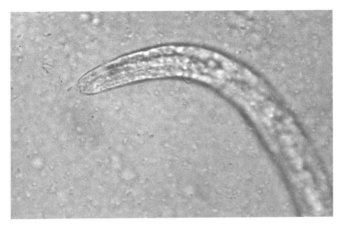

Fig. 154 Strongyloidiasis. *Strongyloides stercoralis* may cause overwhelming autoinfection in patients who are immunocompromised because of leukaemia, lymphoma or treatment with corticosteroids. The rhabditiform larvae of *S. stercoralis* are distinguished from hookworm larvae by the presence of a short buccal capsule.

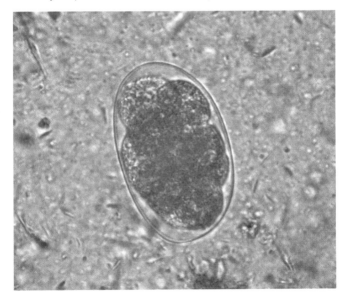

Fig. 155 Hookworm infection. Diagnosis is made by finding the eggs in the faeces. In freshly passed stool specimens the eggs seen are non-embryonated, but if the specimen has been at room temperature for several hours, as in this case, embryos of various stages may be seen within the eggs.

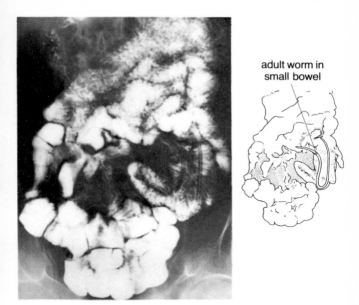

adult worm in
small bowel

Fig. 156   Ascariasis. The large adult worms, which may reach a foot in length, live in the lumen of the small intestine. In this barium study the intestinal tract of one of the adult worms is also well outlined with barium which it has ingested. Most infections are asymptomatic but heavy infection can be associated with malabsorption and malnutrition, or obstruction of the intestine or biliary tract.

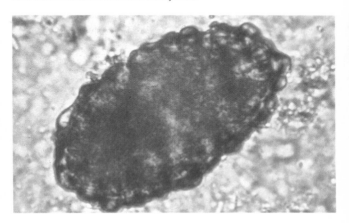

Fig. 157   Ascariasis. Unfertilized eggs of *Ascaris lumbricoides* may be seen in patients harbouring only female worms, and they are occasionally mistaken for vegetable cells. Note the pronounced ellipsoidal shape and indistinct internal structure.

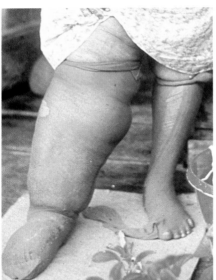

Fig. 158 Bancroftian filariasis. Chronic inflammatory changes in the infected lymphatic system may lead to lymphatic obstruction and elephantiasis of the scrotum or lower extremities, as seen in this woman from Porto Limon, Costa Rica. By courtesy of Dr. R. Muller.

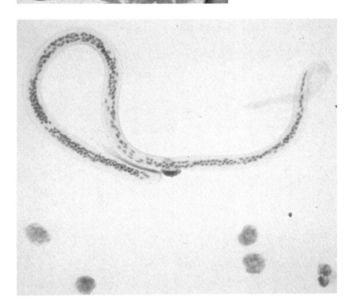

Fig. 159 Bancroftian filariasis. Diagnosis is made by finding the sheathed microfilaria of *Wuchereria bancrofti* in a stained smear of blood taken from the patient around midnight; these may also occasionally be found in hydrocoele fluid or urine. Haematoxylin stain. By courtesy of Dr. R. Muller.

79

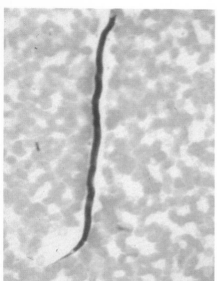

Fig. 160 Loiasis. In this disease the sheathed microfilaria of *Loa loa* are found in the blood during the daytime. Wright's stain. By courtesy of Dr. H. P. Holley, Jr.

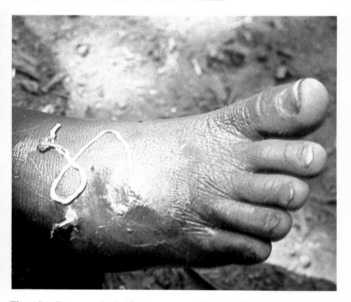

Fig. 161 Dracunculiasis (Guinea worm infection). Contact with water stimulates the adult female Guinea worm *(Dracunculus medinensis)* to emerge from beneath the skin and release large numbers of larvae. As in this case the ulcerated lesion often becomes secondarily infected with bacteria. By courtesy of Dr. R. Muller.

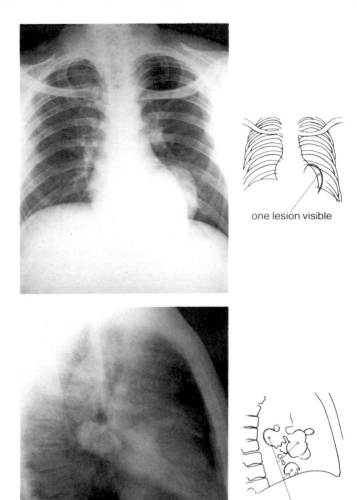

one lesion visible

multiple lesions visible

Fig. 162 Hydatid disease. Man can be an accidental host for the dog tapeworm, *Echinococcus granulosus,* of which the usual intermediate host is sheep or cattle. Hydatid cysts are found most commonly in the liver but can also occur in the lung, brain, bones, peritoneum and in other organs. These radiographs show well-defined rounded cysts in the left lower lobe.

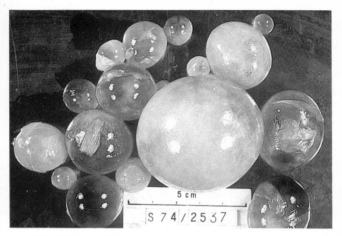

Fig. 163 Echinococcosis. Hydatid cysts are most commonly found in the liver and lung. Rupture of a cyst through the capsule of the liver into the peritoneal cavity results in formation of daughter cysts throughout the peritoneum and omentum, as shown in this surgical specimen.

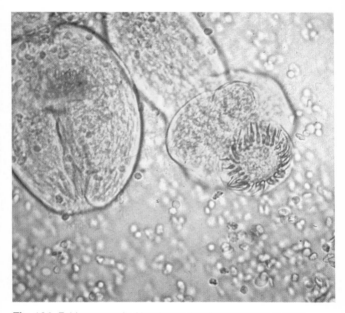

Fig. 164 Echinococcosis. New larvae (scolices) develop in large numbers from the germinal layer of brood capsules within the walls of a cyst. Note both invaginated and evaginated hooklets and suckers. By courtesy of Prof. W. Peters.

82

Index

All entries refer to Fig. numbers